Turkish

Cookbook

77 tasty, delicious, Traditional Recipes from Turkey and the Balkans

By

Ronald M. Dean

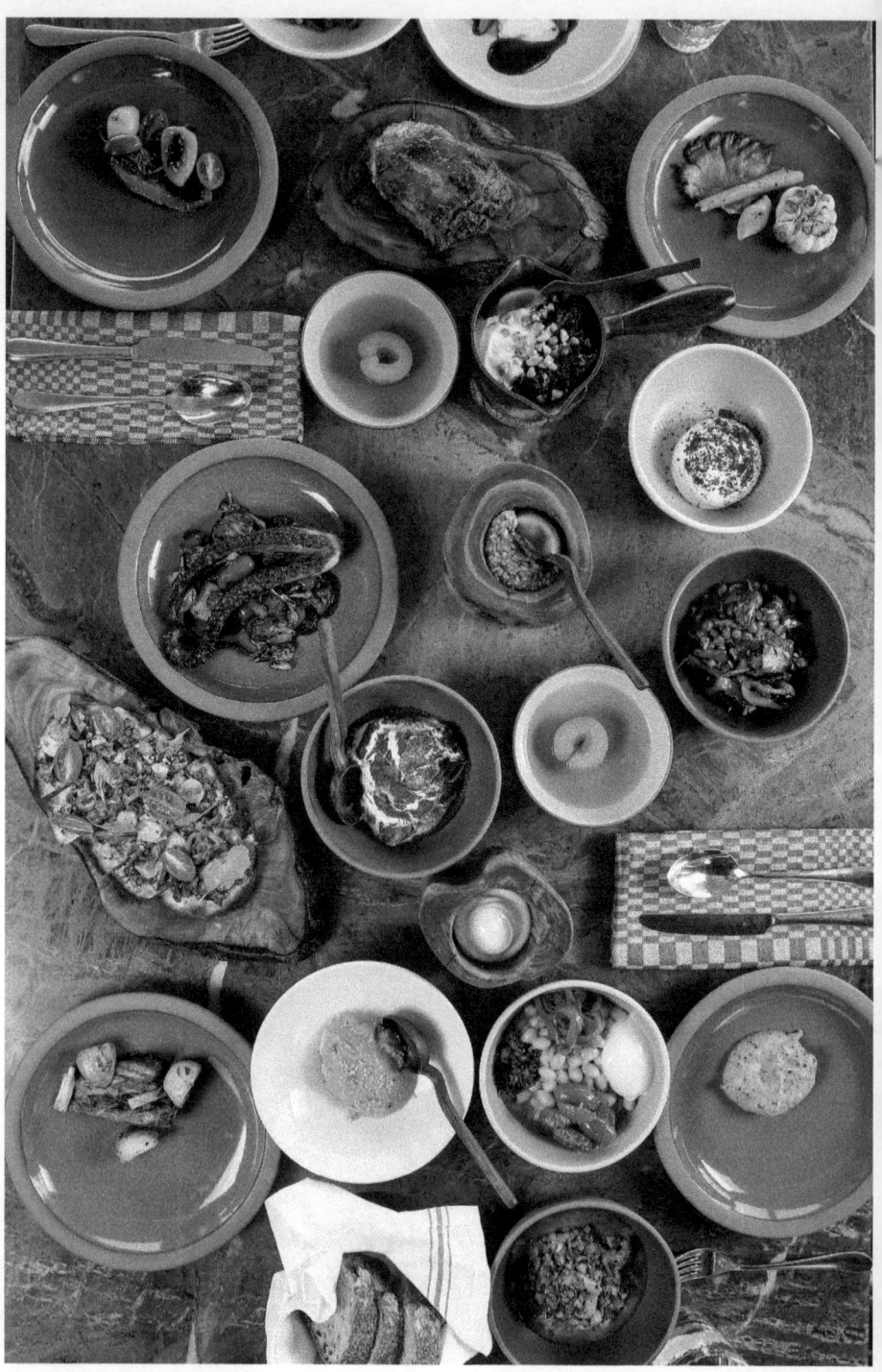

Turkish Cookbook

© Copyright 2021 by Ronald M. Dean- All rights reserved.

This document is geared towards providing exact and reliable information in regard to the topic and issue covered. The publication is sold with the idea that the publisher is not required to render accounting, officially permitted, or otherwise, qualified services. If advice is necessary, legal or professional, a practiced individual in the profession should be ordered.

From a Declaration of Principles which was accepted and approved equally by a Committee of the American Bar Association and a Committee of Publishers and Associations.

In no way is it legal to reproduce, duplicate, or transmit any part of this document in either electronic means or in printed format. Recording of this publication is strictly prohibited and any storage of this document is not allowed unless with written permission from the publisher. All rights reserved.

The information provided herein is stated to be truthful and consistent, in that any liability, in terms of inattention or otherwise, by any usage or abuse of any policies, processes, or directions contained within is the solitary and utter responsibility of the recipient reader. Under no circumstances will any legal responsibility or blame be held against the publisher for any reparation, damages, or monetary loss due to the information herein, either directly or indirectly.

Respective authors own all copyrights not held by the publisher.

The information herein is offered for informational purposes solely and is universal as so. The presentation of the information is without contract or any type of guarantee assurance.

The trademarks that are used are without any consent, and the publication of the trademark is without permission or backing by the trademark owner. All trademarks and brands within this book are for clarifying purposes only and are owned by the owners themselves, not affiliated with this document.

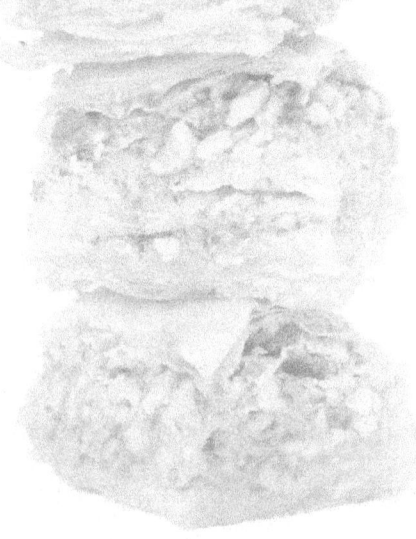

Turkish Cookbook

Table of contents

INTRODUCTION	**8**
CHAPTER 1: WELCOME TO THE WORLD OF TURKISH BREAKFAST RECIPES	**10**
1.1 CILBIR: TURKISH EGGS IN SPICED YOGHURT	10
1.2 YUMURTALI PIDE: TURKISH FLATBREAD	12
1.3 BOYOZ: TURKISH BREAKFAST DISH	13
1.4 TURKISH MENEMEN	14
1.5 BAL KAYMAK	16
1.6 KATMER: TURKISH PANCAKES	17
1.7 GÖZLEME: TURKISH STUFFED BREAD	18
1.8 BÖREK	19
1.9 TURKISH BAGELS	21
1.10 TURKISH SCRAMBLED EGGS	22
1.11 SUCUKLU YUMURTA	24
1.12 TURKISH MIHLAMA	25
1.13 TURKISH BREAKFAST BREAD	26
1.14 TURKISH BAKED EGGS	27
CHAPTER 2: THE WORLD OF TURKISH LUNCH RECIPES	**29**
2.1 TURKISH BEEF MEATBALLS	29
2.2 TURKISH MUHAMMARA	30
2.3 TURKISH STEW	32
2.4 TURKISH MANTI	33
2.5 LAHMACUN: TURKISH PIZZA	34
2.6 KISIR: TURKISH SALAD	36

2.7 COBAN KAVURMA: TURKISH LAMB CASSEROLE   37
2.8 TURKISH KÖFTE   38
2.9 KUMPIR: BAKED POTATOES   40
2.10 BELEN PAN   41
2.11 ADANA KEBAB   42
2.12 TURKISH RICE AND LENTILS   43
2.13 FIRIN MAKARNA: TURKISH MACARONI CHEESE   45
2.16 TURKISH CHICKEN GÖZLEME   46

CHAPTER 3: THE WORLD OF TURKISH DINNER RECIPES   48

3.1 TURKISH MUSAKKA   48
3.2 TURKISH KISIR   49
3.3 TURKISH IMAM BAYILDI   51
3.4 TURKISH MEAT ROLLS   52
3.5 TURKISH BULGAR PILAF   53
3.6 TURKISH KESKEK   54
3.7 TURKISH LENTIL SOUP   55
3.8 TURKISH HALLOUMI BAKE   57
3.9 BARBUNYA PILAKI   58
3.10 CIVIZLI BIBER   59
3.11 TAVUK ŚIŚ   60
3.12 ARNAVUT CIGERI   61
3.13 KARNIYARIK   63

CHAPTER 4: THE WORLD OF TURKISH SNACK RECIPES   65

4.1 TURKISH POGAÇA: DUMPLINGS   65
4.2 TURKISH TULIMBA: FRIED DOUGH   66
4.3 TURKISH SESAME BREAD   67
4.4 TURKISH KABAK TATLISI: PUMPKIN DESSERT   69
4.5 TURKISH SIGARA BOREK   70
4.6 TURKISH DELIGHT   71

Turkish Cookbook

4.7 TURKISH ŚUTLAC	72
4.8 TURKISH CHURROS	73
4.9 TURKISH BAKLAVA	74
4.10 TURKISH COFFEE	75
4.11 TURKISH HELVA	76
4.12 KABAK MÜCVERI: TURKISH FRITTERS	77
4.13 TURKISH HAYDARI	78
4.14 HUMMUS	79

CHAPTER 5: THE WORLD OF TURKISH VEGETARIAN RECIPES
81

5.1 YAPRAK SARMA	81
5.2 ENGINAR KALBI	82
5.3 BARBUNYA: TURKISH BEANS	84
5.4 CARROT BALLS AND YOGHURT	85
5.5 FIRIN SEBZE	86
5.6 KURU FASULYE: TURKISH BEAN STEW	88
5.7 CORBA: TURKISH SOUP	89
5.8 ZEYTINYAGLI TAZE FASULYE	90
5.9 DOLMA	91
5.10 NOHUTLU PILAV: TURKISH RICE WITH CHICKPEAS	93
5.11 TURKISH STUFFED PEPPERS	94
5.12 TURKISH BATRIK	95
5.13 CIG KOFTE	96

CONCLUSION
98

Turkish Cookbook

Introduction

The Turkish and Balkan food depends on the remnants of the Ottoman court and the Greek cooking with an inclination for rice over the bulgur. Less flavors are utilized contrasted with other local Turkish cooking styles, and fish is bountiful and appreciated in any season.

The Turkish and Balkan cuisines are inspiring and exciting for the individuals who travel in culinary pursuits. The assortment of dishes that make up the cuisine, the ways the people meet up in gala like dinners, and the clear unpredictability of each art offer enough material for long investigation and satisfaction.

Turkey is known for a wealth and variety of staple because of its rich greenery, fauna and territorial separation. The tradition of an imperial kitchen is unpreventable. Many cooks spend significant time in making various kinds of dishes, all anxious to satisfy the regal sense of taste, almost certainly had their impact in consummating the cuisine as far as we might be concerned today.

Eggs, fruits and vegetables, dairy and meat are loved all through Turkey and Balkans, guaranteeing profoundly nutritious and crisp tasting food. The flavors and other ingredients that go into Turkish

Cuisine are not just tasty, they have cell reinforcement properties, attempting to bring down cholesterol, dispose of poisons and assist our immunity. Olive oil is customarily used to cook and produce healthy meals, giving cancer prevention agents and fundamental trans fats to your diet. While the presence of fish in the diet adds fundamental unsaturated fats to your eating regimen.

This book contains all the traditional dishes from the Turkey and Balkans that you would love to make on your own. There are 77 various dishes that range from breakfast, lunch, dinners, snacks, and vegetarian recipes that are famous all across the world. So, start reading and start enjoying the amazing taste and aroma of Turkish food at your home!

Chapter 1: Welcome to the World of Turkish Breakfast Recipes

Turkey and Balkans are famous for their amazing, healthy, and unique cuisine. This chapter contains all the famous and traditional breakfast recipes that you have been wanting to make on your own.

1.1 Cilbir: Turkish Eggs in Spiced Yoghurt

Preparation Time: 25 minutes
Cooking Time: 10 minutes
Serving: 2

Ingredients:

- Cayenne pepper, a pinch
- Chopped garlic, two tsp.
- Vinegar, one tbsp.
- Chopped fresh dill, two tbsp.
- Butter, two tbsp.
- Chili flakes, two tbsp.

- Salt to taste
- Black pepper to taste
- Greek yoghurt, one cup
- Eggs, four
- Ground cumin and paprika, one tbsp.

Instructions:
1. Make the spiced yoghurt by mixing in the chopped garlic, fresh dill, and cayenne pepper.
2. Take a saucepan and heat it.
3. When heated add butter into it.
4. Once the butter is hot enough, add the ground cumin and paprika.
5. Add the chili flakes and cook it for two minutes.
6. Take a separate saucepan and add water into it.
7. When boiled properly, add in vinegar.
8. Break the egg into the boiling water.
9. Cook it for five minutes.
10. In the meanwhile, spread the prepared yoghurt on a plate.
11. When eggs are done, add the egg on top of the yoghurt.
12. Spread the prepared butter mixture on top of the egg.
13. Your dish is ready to be served.

1.2 Yumurtali Pide: Turkish Flatbread

Preparation Time: 25 minutes

Cooking Time: 20 minutes

Serving: 4

Ingredients:

- Yeast, two tbsp.
- Sugar, two tsp.
- Green onions, three tbsp.
- Bell pepper strips, half cup
- All-purpose flour, two cups
- Olive oil, two tbsp.
- Vegetable oil, two tbsp.
- Salt to taste
- Black pepper to taste
- Milk, two cups
- Eggs, two
- Mix cheese, two cups
- Water, as required

Instructions:

1. In a bowl mix in the yeast, sugar and two tablespoon water.

2. In a separate bowl add flour, salt, the prepared yeast mixture, and milk.
3. Knead the dough, add olive oil and then let it rise.
4. Once risen, shape it in the form of a pide leaving space in between.
5. Add the chopped green onion, green bell pepper, break in the eggs and spread the mix cheese on top.
6. Add salt and pepper.
7. Let it bake for twenty minutes.
8. Your dish is ready to be served.

1.3 Boyoz: Turkish Breakfast Dish

Preparation Time: 25 minutes
Cooking Time: 30 minutes
Serving: 4

Ingredients:
- Yeast, two tbsp.
- Sugar, two tbsp.
- Parsley, half cup
- All-purpose flour, two cups
- Olive oil, two tbsp.
- Vegetable oil, two tbsp.

- Salt to taste
- Black pepper to taste
- Milk, two cups
- Mix cheese, two cups
- Water, as required

Instructions:
1. In a bowl, mix in the yeast, sugar and two tablespoon water.
2. In a separate bowl, add flour, salt, the prepared yeast mixture, and milk.
3. Knead the dough, add olive oil and then let it rise.
4. Make small round balls out of the dough.
5. Mix the cheese and parsley.
6. Fill these balls with the cheese and parsley mixture above.
7. Cover it with olive oil and bake for twenty to twenty-five minutes.
8. Your dish is ready to be served.

1.4 Turkish Menemen

Preparation Time: 5 minutes
Cooking Time: 10 minutes
Serving: 4

Ingredients:

- Olive oil, two tbsp.
- Chopped garlic, two tsp.
- Tomatoes, three tbsp.
- Bell pepper strips, half cup
- Chopped fresh dill, two tbsp.
- Parsley, two tbsp.
- Salt to taste
- Black pepper to taste
- Eggs, four
- Chopped onions, two tbsp.

Instructions:

1. In a pan add the olive oil and onion.
2. Cook the onions until they are soft.
3. Add the garlic into it and cook.
4. Add in the bell pepper strips and tomatoes.
5. Add salt and pepper to taste.
6. Add in the fresh chopped dill.
7. When the mixture is ready, break in the eggs all over the mixture.
8. Do not mix it but cover it for ten minutes on low heat.
9. After ten minutes, add in the parsley.
10. Your dish is ready to be served.

1.5 Bal Kayamak

Preparation Time: 10 minutes
Cooking Time: 3 hours
Serving: 6

Ingredients:

- Heavy cream, three cups
- Milk, four cups
- Salt, two tsp.

Instructions:

1. Take a deep dish and add milk into it.
2. Let the milk boil and then add the heavy cream into the mixture.
3. Add in the salt.
4. Keep mixing the milk and cream for one hour and then let it cool down.
5. After it cools down, place it back on the heat.
6. Simmer it more for two hour and then place it in the refrigerator for two hours.
7. Your dish is ready to be served.

1.6 Katmer: Turkish Pancakes

Preparation Time: 25 minutes

Cooking Time: 15 minutes

Serving: 4

Ingredients:
- Honey, two tbsp.
- Puff pastry dough, a pack
- Pistachio, three tbsp.
- Clotted cream, half cup
- Sugar, two tbsp.
- Unsalted butter, two tbsp.

Instructions:
1. Add two pastry sheets on top of another on a dry surface.
2. Spread little amount of the cream all around the pastry sheet.
3. Sprinkle the finely squashed pistachios and sugar uniformly over the cream.
4. Add the leftover sheets on top.
5. Cut them into little squares.
6. Brush the edges of the top pastry with softened spread.
7. Take a pan and heat it well.

8. Add the pastry into the pan and cook for two minutes.
9. Turn them over delicately and cook for an additional minute or two.
10. Serve the katmer warm, showered with honey.
11. Your dish is ready to be served.

1.7 Gözleme: Turkish Stuffed Bread

Preparation Time: 25 minutes
Cooking Time: 30 minutes
Serving: 4

Ingredients:

- Yeast, two tbsp.
- Sugar, two tbsp.
- Parsley, half cup
- Minced beef, one pound
- Tomatoes, half cup
- All-purpose flour, two cups
- Olive oil, two tbsp.
- Vegetable oil, two tbsp.
- Salt to taste
- Black pepper to taste
- Milk, two cups

- Mix cheese, two cups
- Water, as required

Instructions:
1. In a bowl mix in the yeast, sugar and two tablespoon water.
2. In a separate bowl add flour, salt, the prepared yeast mixture, and milk.
3. Knead the dough, add olive oil and then let it rise.
4. Make small round balls out of the dough.
5. In a pan add the olive oil, tomatoes, and beef and let it cook.
6. When it is cooked, cool it down.
7. Make flat bread from these balls.
8. Fill this bread with the cheese and parsley and the beef mixture above.
9. Cover it with olive oil and bake for twenty to twenty-five minutes.
10. Your dish is ready to be served.

1.8 Börek

Preparation Time: 25 minutes

Cooking Time: 15 minutes

Serving: 4

Ingredients:

- Honey, two tbsp.
- Puff pastry dough, a pack
- Egg, one
- Yoghurt, half cup
- Sugar, two tbsp.
- Unsalted butter, two tbsp.

Instructions:

1. Mix the egg, yoghurt, sugar, butter, and honey together.
2. Add two pastry sheets on top of another on a dry surface.
3. Spread little amount of the mixture all around the pastry sheet.
4. Add the leftover sheets on top.
5. Cut them into little squares.
6. Brush the edges of the top pastry with softened spread.
7. Take a pan and heat it well.
8. Add the pastry into the oven and cook for forty minutes.
9. Serve the borek warm.
10. Your dish is ready to be served.

1.9 Turkish Bagels

Preparation Time: 25 minutes

Cooking Time: 15 minutes

Serving: 4

Ingredients:

- Yeast, two tbsp.
- Sugar, two tbsp.
- Molasses, half cup
- All-purpose flour, two cups
- Olive oil, two tbsp.
- Sesame seeds, two tbsp.
- Egg, one
- Warm water, two cups

Instructions:

1. In a bowl, mix in the yeast, sugar and two tablespoon water.
2. In a separate bowl, add flour, salt, the prepared yeast mixture, and milk.
3. Knead the dough, add olive oil and then let it rise.
4. Make small bagels out of the dough.
5. Mix the molasses and sesame seeds.

6. Dip the bagels in the sesame seeds mixture and place it on a baking dish.
7. Cover it with egg wash and bake for twenty to twenty-five minutes.
8. Your dish is ready to be served.

1.10 Turkish Scrambled Eggs

Preparation Time: 25 minutes
Cooking Time: 15 minutes
Serving: 4

Ingredients:
- Chopped garlic, two tsp.
- Green onions, three tbsp.
- Bell pepper strips, two cups
- Chopped fresh dill, two tbsp.
- Vegetable oil, two tbsp.
- Salt to taste
- Black pepper to taste
- Eggs, six
- Chopped onions, two tbsp.

Instructions:
1. In a bowl, whisk together salt, eggs, and pepper.
2. Add vegetable oil.
3. Add the onion and blend well.
4. Spread into a solitary layer and cook for thirty seconds.
5. Add in the garlic paste.
6. Include the peppers.
7. When cooked, push vegetables to a corner.
8. Mix in the egg combination and whirl delicately to spread around skillet.
9. Delicately but rapidly mix constantly to scramble eggs.
10. Mix vegetables into eggs as you scramble them.
11. At the point when eggs are simply cooked, but not dry, eliminate them from the heat.
12. Add the green onions, dill and blend well.
13. Your dish is ready to be served.

1.11 Sucuklu Yumurta

Preparation Time: 25 minutes
Cooking Time: 15 minutes
Serving: 4

Ingredients:

- Chopped garlic, two tsp.
- Green onions, three tbsp.
- Sucuk, two cups
- Chopped fresh dill, two tbsp.
- Vegetable oil, two tbsp.
- Salt to taste
- Black pepper to taste
- Eggs, six
- Chopped onions, two tbsp.

Instructions:

1. In a bowl, whisk together salt, eggs, and pepper.
2. Add vegetable oil.
3. Add the onion and blend well.
4. Spread into a solitary layer and cook for thirty seconds.
5. Add in the garlic paste.
6. Include the sucuk.

7. When cooked, push vegetables to a corner.
8. Mix in the egg combination and whirl delicately to spread around skillet.
9. Delicately but rapidly mix constantly to scramble eggs.
10. Mix vegetables into eggs as you scramble them.
11. At the point when eggs are simply cooked, yet not dry, eliminate them from the heat.
12. Add the green onions, dill and blend well.
13. Your dish is ready to be served.

1.12 Turkish Mihlama

Preparation Time: 10 minutes
Cooking Time: 3 hours
Serving: 6

Ingredients:
- Corn flour, one tbsp.
- Water, one tbsp.
- Salt, one tsp.
- Grated kashari cheese, three cups
- Butter, one tbsp.

Instructions:
1. Take a deep dish and add cheese into it.
2. Let the cheese melt and then add the water into the mixture.
3. Add in the salt.
4. Keep mixing the cheese for two minutes.
5. Add the corn flour and butter.
6. Mix the cheese until it forms into a smooth mixture.
7. Your dish is ready to be served.

1.13 Turkish Breakfast Bread

Preparation Time: 25 minutes

Cooking Time: 20 minutes

Serving: 4

Ingredients:
- Yeast, two tbsp.
- Sugar, two tsp.
- All-purpose flour, two cups
- Olive oil, two tbsp.
- Vegetable oil, two tbsp.
- Milk, two cups
- Water, as required

Instructions:
1. In a bowl mix in the yeast, sugar and two tablespoon water.
2. In a separate bowl add flour, salt, the prepared yeast mixture, and milk.
3. Knead the dough, add olive oil and then let it rise.
4. Once risen, shape it in the form of a loaf.
5. Let it bake for twenty minutes.
6. Once baked you can serve it with various things in the morning.
7. Your dish is ready to be served.

1.14 Turkish Baked Eggs

Preparation Time: 5 minutes
Cooking Time: 10 minutes
Serving: 4

Ingredients:
- Olive oil, two tbsp.
- Chopped garlic, two tsp.
- Tomatoes, three tbsp.
- Bell pepper strips, half cup
- Chopped fresh dill, two tbsp.
- Parsley, two tbsp.

- Salt to taste
- Black pepper to taste
- Eggs, four
- Corn kernels, half cup
- Chopped onions, two tbsp.
- Bread slices, as required

Instructions:
1. In a pan, add the olive oil and onion.
2. Cook the onions until they are soft.
3. Add the garlic into it and cook.
4. Add in the bell pepper strips and tomatoes.
5. Add in the corn kernels.
6. Add salt and pepper to taste.
7. Add in the fresh chopped dill.
8. When the mixture is ready, break in the eggs all over the mixture.
9. Do not mix it.
10. Bake it for ten minutes on low heat.
11. After ten minutes add in the parsley.
12. Serve with bread slices.
13. Your dish is ready to be served.

Chapter 2: The World of Turkish Lunch Recipes

This chapter contains all the famous and traditional lunch recipes that you have been wanting to make on your own.

2.1 Turkish Beef Meatballs

Preparation Time: 25 minutes
Cooking Time: 30 minutes
Serving: 4

Ingredients:
- Mix Turkish spice, two tbsp.
- Chopped garlic, two tsp.
- Green onions, three tbsp.
- Minced beef, two cups
- Chopped fresh dill, two tbsp.
- Vegetable oil, half cup
- Salt to taste
- Black pepper to taste
- Bread crumbs, two tbsp.
- Eggs, one
- Chopped onions, two tbsp.

Instructions:

1. In a bowl, add the minced beef, chopped garlic, onions, fresh dill, spices, bread crumbs, eggs, together.
2. Mix the above ingredients to form a fine and smooth structure.
3. Make small round ball like structures.
4. In a pan, add the oil and heat it.
5. When the oil is heated enough, add the meatballs and fry them all over.
6. When the meatballs are golden brown in color, dish them out.
7. Your dish is ready to be served.

2.2 Turkish Muhammara

Preparation Time: 20 minutes
Cooking Time: 30 minutes
Serving: 6

Ingredients:

- Pomegranate juice, two tbsp.
- Chopped garlic, two tsp.
- Bread crumbs, three tbsp.

- Bell pepper strips, four cups
- Walnuts, two cups
- Chopped fresh dill, two tbsp.
- Vegetable oil, two tbsp.
- Lemon juice, two tbsp.
- Salt to taste
- Black pepper to taste
- Paprika, one tsp.
- Cumin seeds, one tsp.
- Chili flakes, two tbsp.

Instructions:
1. Slice the bell pepper and drizzle some oil on top.
2. Place the bell pepper in the oven for five to ten minutes until they become soft.
3. When the bell peppers become soft and crunchy take them out of the oven.
4. In a blender add the chopped garlic, bell pepper, lemon juice, paprika, cumin seeds, chili flakes, walnuts, fresh dill, pomegranate juice, and bread crumbs.
5. Make a smooth paste from the ingredients above.
6. Add in the salt and pepper to taste.
7. Your dish is ready to be served.

2.3 Turkish Stew

Preparation Time: 25 minutes
Cooking Time: 40 minutes
Serving: 4

Ingredients:

- Mix Turkish spice, two tbsp.
- Chopped garlic, two tsp.
- Green onions, three tbsp.
- Beef chunks, two cups
- Beef stock, three cups
- Chopped fresh dill, two tbsp.
- Vegetable oil, half cup
- Salt to taste
- Black pepper to taste
- Parsley, two tbsp.
- Tomatoes, one cup
- Chopped onions, two tbsp.

Instructions:

1. Add the oil in a deep pan.
2. Add the chopped onions when the oil is hot.
3. When the onions are soft enough, add the garlic into it.

4. Add in the tomatoes and all the spices.
5. Add in the beef chunks and mix it for ten minutes.
6. Add in the beef stock and let the stew simmer for thirty minutes.
7. In the end, add the green onions and parsley and dish out.
8. Your dish is ready to be served.

2.4 Turkish Manti

Preparation Time: 25 minutes
Cooking Time: 10 minutes
Serving: 2

Ingredients:
- Cayenne pepper, a pinch
- Chopped garlic, two tsp.
- Vinegar, one tbsp.
- Chopped fresh dill, two tbsp.
- Butter, two tbsp.
- Chili flakes, two tbsp.
- Salt to taste
- Black pepper to taste
- Greek yoghurt, one cup
- Dumplings, one pound

- Ground cumin and paprika, one tbsp.

Instructions:
1. Make the spiced yoghurt by mixing in the chopped garlic, fresh dill, and cayenne pepper.
2. Take a saucepan and heat it.
3. When heated, add butter into it.
4. Once the butter is hot enough, add the ground cumin and paprika.
5. Add the chili flakes and cook it for two minutes.
6. Take a separate saucepan and add water into it.
7. When boiled to the right amount add in vinegar.
8. Add in the dumplings into the boiling water.
9. Cook it for five minutes.
10. In the meanwhile, spread the prepared yoghurt on a plate.
11. When the dumplings are done add the dumplings on top of the yoghurt.
12. Spread the prepared butter mixture on top of the dumplings.
13. Your dish is ready to be served.

2.5 Lahmacun: Turkish Pizza

Preparation Time: 25 minutes

Cooking Time: 20 minutes

Serving: 4

Ingredients:
- Yeast, two tbsp.
- Sugar, two tsp.
- Bell pepper strips, half cup
- All-purpose flour, two cups
- Olive oil, two tbsp.
- Olives, half cup
- Vegetable oil, two tbsp.
- Salt to taste
- Black pepper to taste
- Milk, two cups
- Cooked beef mince, one cup
- Mix cheese, two cups
- Water, as required

Instructions:
1. In a bowl, mix in the yeast, sugar and two tablespoon water.
2. In a separate bowl, add flour, salt, the prepared yeast mixture, and milk.
3. Knead the dough, add olive oil and then let it rise.
4. Once risen, shape it in the form of a pizza.

5. Add the chopped green onion, green bell pepper, prepared meat, olives and spread the mix cheese on top.
6. Add salt and pepper.
7. Let it bake for twenty minutes.
8. Your dish is ready to be served.

2.6 Kisir: Turkish Salad

Preparation Time: 25 minutes
Cooking Time: 5 minutes
Serving Size: 4-6

Ingredients:
- Shredded green cabbage, two cups
- Cooked bulgar, two cups
- Sliced red bell pepper, one cup
- Shredded carrots, one cup
- Sliced yellow bell pepper, one cup
- Green onions, a quarter cup
- Honey, two tbsp.
- Parsley, a quarter cup
- Salt and pepper to taste
- Sesame seeds, half cup

Instructions:
1. Add all of the salad ingredients to a large bowl.
2. Drizzle your desired amount of the sesame seeds over the salad.
3. Toss the salad until well combined.
4. Your dish is ready to be served.

2.7 Coban Kavurma: Turkish Lamb Casserole

Preparation Time: 25 minutes
Cooking Time: 30 minutes
Serving: 4

Ingredients:
- Mix Turkish spice, two tbsp.
- Chopped garlic, two tsp.
- Green onions, three tbsp.
- Minced beef, two cups
- Chopped fresh dill, two tbsp.
- Vegetable oil, half cup
- Salt to taste
- Black pepper to taste
- Bread crumbs, two tbsp.
- Eggs, two

- Chopped onions, two tbsp.
- Mix cheese, one cup

Instructions:
1. In a bowl, add the minced beef, chopped garlic, onions, fresh dill, spices, bread crumbs together.
2. Mix the above ingredients to form a fine and smooth structure.
3. Add the mixture into a baking dish.
4. Add in eggs and mix properly.
5. Spread the cheese on top and bake.
6. When the cheese turns golden brown dish out.
7. Your dish is ready to be served.

2.8 Turkish Köfte

Preparation Time: 25 minutes
Cooking Time: 30 minutes
Serving: 4

Ingredients:
- Mix Turkish spice, two tbsp.
- Chopped garlic, two tsp.
- Green onions, three tbsp.

Turkish Cookbook

- Minced beef, two cups
- Chopped fresh dill, two tbsp.
- Vegetable oil, half cup
- Salt to taste
- Black pepper to taste
- Bread crumbs, two tbsp.
- Eggs, one
- Chopped onions, two tbsp.
- Tomato puree, two cups

Instructions:
1. In a bowl, add the minced beef, chopped garlic, onions, fresh dill, spices, bread crumbs, eggs, together.
2. Mix the above ingredients to form a fine and smooth structure.
3. Make small round ball like structures.
4. Add the oil in a pan and heat it.
5. When the oil is heated enough, add the meatballs and fry them all over.
6. When the meatballs are golden brown in color dish them out.
7. In a pan add the tomato puree and place the meatballs in it.
8. Once the gravy is cooked switch off the stove.
9. Your dish is ready to be served.

Turkish Cookbook

2.9 Kumpir: Baked Potatoes

Preparation Time: 25 minutes
Cooking Time: 30 minutes
Serving: 4

Ingredients:
- Mix Turkish spice, two tbsp.
- Chopped garlic, two tsp.
- Green onions, three tbsp.
- Potato cubes, two cups
- Chopped fresh dill, two tbsp.
- Vegetable oil, half cup
- Salt to taste
- Black pepper to taste
- Chopped onions, two tbsp.
- Mix cheese, one cup

Instructions:
1. In a bowl, add the potato cubes, chopped garlic, onions, fresh dill, spices together.
2. Drizzle oil on top of the potatoes.
3. Place it in a baking dish.

4. Add the shredded cheese on top.
5. Bake for ten to fifteen minutes.
6. Your dish is ready to be served.

2.10 Belen Pan

Preparation Time: 25 minutes
Cooking Time: 40 minutes
Serving: 4

Ingredients:
- Mix Turkish spice, two tbsp.
- Chopped garlic, two tsp.
- Green onions, three tbsp.
- Beef chunks, two cups
- Mix vegetables, two cups
- Chopped fresh dill, two tbsp.
- Vegetable oil, half cup
- Salt to taste
- Black pepper to taste
- Parsley, two tbsp.
- Tomatoes, one cup
- Chopped onions, two tbsp.

Instructions:
1. Add the oil in a deep pan.
2. Add the chopped onions when the oil is hot.
3. When the onions are soft enough, add the garlic into it.
4. Add in the tomatoes and all the spices.
5. Add in the beef chunks and mix it for ten minutes.
6. Add in the mixed vegetables and let it cook for thirty minutes.
7. In the end, add the green onions and parsley and dish out.
8. Your dish is ready to be served.

2.11 Adana Kebab

Preparation Time: 25 minutes
Cooking Time: 30 minutes
Serving: 4

Ingredients:
- Mix Turkish spice, two tbsp.
- Chopped garlic, two tsp.
- Green onions, three tbsp.
- Minced lamb, two cups
- Chopped fresh dill, two tbsp.
- Vegetable oil, half cup

- Salt to taste
- Black pepper to taste
- Bread crumbs, two tbsp.
- Eggs, one
- Chopped onions, two tbsp.

Instructions:
1. In a bowl, add the minced lamb, chopped garlic, onions, fresh dill, spices, bread crumbs, eggs, together.
2. Mix the above ingredients to form a fine and smooth structure.
3. Make long finger like structures.
4. In a pan, add the oil and heat it.
5. When the oil is heated enough, add the kebab and fry them all over.
6. When the kebabs are golden brown in color dish them out.
7. Your dish is ready to be served.

2.12 Turkish Rice and Lentils

Preparation Time: 25 minutes

Cooking Time: 40 minutes

Serving: 4

Ingredients:

- Mix Turkish spice, two tbsp.
- Chopped garlic, two tsp.
- Green onions, three tbsp.
- Lentils, two cups
- Rice, three cups
- Chopped fresh dill, two tbsp.
- Vegetable oil, half cup
- Salt to taste
- Black pepper to taste
- Parsley, two tbsp.
- Tomatoes, one cup
- Chopped onions, two tbsp.

Instructions:

1. Add the oil in a deep pan.
2. Add the chopped onions when the oil is hot.
3. When the onions are soft enough, add the garlic into it.
4. Add in the tomatoes and all the spices.
5. Add in the lentils and mix it for ten minutes.
6. Add in the rice and let the stew simmer for thirty minutes.
7. In the end, add the green onions and parsley and dish out.
8. Your dish is ready to be served.

2.13 Firin Makarna: Turkish Macaroni Cheese

Preparation Time: 25 minutes

Cooking Time: 30 minutes

Serving: 4

Ingredients:

- Mix Turkish spice, two tbsp.
- Chopped garlic, two tsp.
- Green onions, three tbsp.
- Cooked macaroni, two cups
- Chopped fresh dill, two tbsp.
- Vegetable oil, half cup
- Salt to taste
- Black pepper to taste
- Chopped onions, two tbsp.
- White sauce, two cups
- Mix cheese, one cup

Instructions:

1. In a bowl, add the boiled macaroni, chopped garlic, onions, fresh dill, spices together.
2. Add the white sauce on top of the above mixture.
3. Place it in a baking dish.

4. Add the shredded cheese on top.
5. Bake for ten to fifteen minutes.
6. Your dish is ready to be served.

2.16 Turkish Chicken Gözleme

Preparation Time: 25 minutes
Cooking Time: 30 minutes
Serving: 4

Ingredients:
- Yeast, two tbsp.
- Sugar, two tbsp.
- Parsley, half cup
- Minced chicken, one pound
- Tomatoes, half cup
- All-purpose flour, two cups
- Olive oil, two tbsp.
- Vegetable oil, two tbsp.
- Salt to taste
- Black pepper to taste
- Milk, two cups
- Mix cheese, two cups
- Water, as required

Instructions:

1. In a bowl, mix in the yeast, sugar and two tablespoon water.
2. In a separate bowl, add flour, salt, the prepared yeast mixture, and milk.
3. Knead the dough, add olive oil and then let it rise.
4. Make small round balls out of the dough.
5. In a pan, add the olive oil, tomatoes, and chicken and let it cook.
6. When cooked, cool it down.
7. Make flat bread from these balls.
8. Fill this bread with the cheese and parsley and the chicken mixture above.
9. Cover it with olive oil and bake for twenty to twenty-five minutes.
10. Your dish is ready to be served.

Chapter 3: The World of Turkish Dinner Recipes

This chapter contains all the famous and traditional dinner recipes that you have been wanting to make on your own.

3.1 Turkish Musakka

Preparation Time: 25 minutes
Cooking Time: 15 minutes
Serving: 4

Ingredients:

- Olive oil, four tbsp.
- Aborigine, cubes
- Green peppers, chopped.
- Bell pepper strips, half cup.
- Tomato paste, two tbsp.
- Tomatoes, chopped.
- Garlic, chopped.
- Beef, 400 g
- Salt to taste
- Black pepper to taste
- Flat leaf parsley, chopped

- Chopped onions, two tbsp.

Instructions:
1. Preheat your oven.
2. Mix aborigine cubes, olive oil, salt, pepper well and then roast until it becomes soft and brownish in color.
3. Heat a fry pan, and brown the beef in olive oil.
4. Fry the onion, green pepper, with salt.
5. Add garlic, tomato paste, sugar and stir it well.
6. Add tomatoes, pepper, and beef and boil them in water until tomatoes are cooked.
7. Add roast aborigine and flat-leaf parsley.
8. Your dish is ready to be served.

3.2 Turkish Kisir

Preparation Time: 25 minutes
Cooking Time: 15 minutes
Serving: 4

Ingredients:
- Dry Bulgur, one cup.
- Chicken broth, half cup.
- Mint, half tbsp.

- Cumin, half tbsp.
- Fresh parsley.
- Red pepper, half tbsp.
- Tomato, two.
- Tomato paste, two tbsp.
- Pepper paste, one tbsp.
- Cucumber, two.
- Green onion, five.
- Lemon juice, two tbsp.
- Olive oil, two or three tbsp.
- Bell pepper strips, half cup.
- Salt to taste.

Instructions:
1. Add the oil in a deep pan.
2. Add the chopped onions when the oil is hot.
3. When the onions are soft enough add the garlic into it.
4. Add in the tomato paste and all the spices.
5. Add in the bulgar and mix it for ten minutes.
6. Add in the pepper paste as well as vegetables.
7. Add in the chicken broth and let the stew simmer for thirty minutes.
8. In the end, add the green onions and parsley along with other remaining ingredients.

9. Your dish is ready to be served.

3.3 Turkish Imam Bayildi

Preparation Time: 25 minutes

Cooking Time: 2 hours

Serving: 4

Ingredients:
- Olive oil, half cup.
- Water, half cup.
- Sugar, three tbsp.
- Chopped garlic, two tsp.
- Eggplants, four
- Bell pepper strips, half cup
- Fresh parsley, chopped.
- Salt to taste
- Black pepper to taste
- Chopped onions, two tbsp.

Instructions:
1. Preheat your oven.
2. Cut the eggplants.
3. Bake for twenty minutes.

4. Remove from oven and allow drying for thirty minutes.
5. Heat olive oil, add the onions.
6. Cook for five to eight minutes.
7. Add garlic, cook and stir for thirty seconds.
8. Add all spices and tomato paste.
9. Take eggplants, fill them with onion and tomato mixture
10. Add lemon juice and sugar as required.
11. Cook eggplants for one to one and half hour.
12. Cool the eggplants.
13. Your dish is ready to be served.

3.4 Turkish Meat Rolls

Preparation Time: 20 minutes

Cooking Time: 25 minutes

Serving: 4

Ingredients:
- Ground lamb, three by four pounds.
- Chopped garlic, two tbsp.
- Phyllo dough, eight sheets.
- Cheese, three by four pounds.
- Parsley, half cup
- Olive oil, one by four cup

- Thyme pepper to taste

Instructions:
1. Brown the meat and add in a bowl.
2. Add parsley, garlic, and pepper.
3. Set aside for twenty-five minutes.
4. Take one sheet of phyllo and spray with olive oil.
5. Brush with egg wash.
6. Fry meat rolls turning to brown.
7. Serve with sauce.
8. Your dish is ready to be served.

3.5 Turkish Bulgar Pilaf

Preparation Time: 25 minutes
Cooking Time: 15 minutes
Serving: 4

Ingredients:
- Bulgur, two cups
- Chopped garlic, two tsp.
- Green onions, three tbsp.
- Bell pepper strips, half cup
- Chopped fresh dill, two tbsp.

- Vegetable oil, two tbsp.
- Soy sauce, two tbsp.
- Salt to taste
- Black pepper to taste
- Eggs, six
- Chopped onions, two tbsp.

Instructions:
1. Heat oil and add bulgur and cook it.
2. Add onion, garlic, green pepper and mix well.
3. Then add all spices to taste.
4. Add tomato and mesh all the ingredients.
5. Cook well for ten minutes.
6. Your dish is ready to be served.

3.6 Turkish Keskek

Preparation Time: 25 minutes

Cooking Time: 15 minutes

Serving: 4

Ingredients:
- Eggplants, two
- Tomato paste.

Turkish Cookbook

- Mint, dried.
- Salt and pepper to taste

Instructions:
1. Peel eggplants and cut them in equal pieces.
2. Then cook it on the stove.
3. Mix tomato paste with water.
4. Brown the onion and fry dried mint
5. Pour the mint over cooked eggplant.
6. Serve your dish.

3.7 Turkish Lentil Soup

Preparation Time: 25 minutes
Cooking Time: 40 minutes
Serving: 4

Ingredients:
- Mix Turkish spice, two tbsp.
- Chopped garlic, two tsp.
- Green onions, three tbsp.
- Lentils, two cups
- Water, two cups
- Corn flour, two tbsp.

- Cooked bulgar, one cup
- Chopped fresh dill, two tbsp.
- Vegetable oil, half cup
- Salt to taste
- Black pepper to taste
- Parsley, two tbsp.
- Tomatoes, one cup
- Chopped onions, two tbsp.

Instructions:
1. Add the oil in a deep pan.
2. Add the chopped onions when the oil is hot.
3. When the onions are soft enough, add the garlic into it.
4. Add in the tomatoes and all the spices.
5. Add in the lentils and mix it for ten minutes.
6. Let the lentils simmer for thirty minutes.
7. Add in the water and cook for five minutes.
8. Add in the corn flour and cooked bulgar.
9. In the end add the green onions and parsley and dish out.
10. Your dish is ready to be served.

3.8 Turkish Halloumi Bake

Preparation Time: 25 minutes

Cooking Time: 30 minutes

Serving: 4

Ingredients:
- Mix Turkish spice, two tbsp.
- Chopped garlic, two tsp.
- Green onions, three tbsp.
- Aborigine cubes, two cups
- Chopped fresh dill, two tbsp.
- Vegetable oil, half cup
- Salt to taste
- Black pepper to taste
- Chopped onions, two tbsp.
- Mix cheese, one cup

Instructions:
1. In a bowl, add the aborigine cubes, chopped garlic, onions, fresh dill, and spices together.
2. Drizzle oil on top of the potatoes.
3. Place it in a baking dish.
4. Add the shredded cheese on top.

5. Bake for ten to fifteen minutes.
6. Your dish is ready to be served.

3.9 Barbunya Pilaki

Preparation Time: 25 minutes
Cooking Time: 40 minutes
Serving: 4

Ingredients:
- Mix Turkish spice, two tbsp.
- Chopped garlic, two tsp.
- Green onions, three tbsp.
- Beans, two cups
- Carrots, two cups
- Vegetable stock, half cup
- Chopped fresh dill, two tbsp.
- Vegetable oil, half cup
- Salt to taste
- Black pepper to taste
- Parsley, two tbsp.
- Tomatoes, one cup
- Chopped onions, two tbsp.

Instructions:

1. Add the oil in a deep pan.
2. Add the chopped onions when the oil is hot.
3. When the onions are soft enough, add the garlic into it.
4. Add in the tomatoes, carrots and all the spices.
5. Add in the beans and mix it for ten minutes.
6. Add in the vegetable stock.
7. Let the mixture simmer for thirty minutes.
8. In the end, add the green onions and parsley and dish out.
9. Your dish is ready to be served.

3.10 Civizli Biber

Preparation Time: 25 minutes

Cooking Time: 15 minutes

Serving: 4

Ingredients:

- Red pepper, one cup
- Walnuts, one cup
- Olive oil, half cup
- Grains, one cup
- Vegetables, cup
- Salt to taste

- Black pepper to taste

Instructions:
1. Take walnuts and fry them.
2. Make paste of all ingredients.
3. Mix it with walnuts.
4. Take it out in a bowl and put some pepper.
5. Add salt to taste.
6. Your dish is ready to be served.

3.11 Tavuk Śiś

Preparation Time: 25 minutes
Cooking Time: 30 minutes
Serving: 4

Ingredients:
- Mix Turkish spice, two tbsp.
- Chopped garlic, two tsp.
- Green onions, three tbsp.
- Minced chicken, two cups
- Chopped fresh dill, two tbsp.
- Vegetable oil, half cup
- Salt to taste

- Black pepper to taste
- Bread crumbs, two tbsp.
- Eggs, one
- Chopped onions, two tbsp.

Instructions:
1. In a bowl, add the minced chicken, chopped garlic, onions, fresh dill, spices, bread crumbs, eggs, together.
2. Mix the above ingredients to form a fine and smooth mixture.
3. Make long finger like structures.
4. In a pan, add the oil and heat it.
5. When the oil is heated enough, add the kebab and fry them all over.
6. When the kebabs are golden brown in color, dish them out.
7. Your dish is ready to be served.

3.12 Arnavut Cigeri

Preparation Time: 25 minutes
Cooking Time: 40 minutes
Serving: 4

Ingredients:

- Mix Turkish spice, two tbsp.
- Chopped garlic, two tsp.
- Green onions, three tbsp.
- Beef chunks, two cups
- Beef stock, three cups
- Chopped fresh dill, two tbsp.
- Vegetable oil, half cup
- Salt to taste
- Black pepper to taste
- Parsley, two tbsp.
- Tomatoes, one cup
- Chopped onions, two tbsp.

Instructions:
1. Add the oil in a deep pan.
2. Add the chopped onions when the oil is hot.
3. When the onions are soft enough, add the garlic into it.
4. Add in the tomatoes and all the spices.
5. Add in the lamb and veal chunks and mix it for ten minutes.
6. Let the lamb and veal chunks simmer for thirty minutes.
7. In the end, add the green onions and parsley and dish out.
8. Your dish is ready to be served.

3.13 Karniyarik

Preparation Time: 25 minutes

Cooking Time: 15 minutes

Serving: 4

Ingredients:
- Olive oil, two tbsp.
- Chopped garlic, two tsp.
- Green onions, three tbsp.
- Eggplant, four
- Zucchini, two cups
- Chopped fresh dill, two tbsp.
- Vegetable oil, two tbsp.
- Salt to taste
- Black pepper to taste
- Bulgar, one cup
- Mixed cheese, one cup
- Chopped onions, two tbsp.

Instructions:
1. Mix all the ingredients together in a bowl.
2. Cut the eggplant in half.
3. Remove the seeds from inside.

Turkish Cookbook

4. Stuff the formed mixture into the eggplant.
5. Place the eggplants on a baking dish.
6. Add the cheese on top.
7. Drizzle oil on top.
8. Bake for fifteen minutes.
9. Your dish is ready to be served.

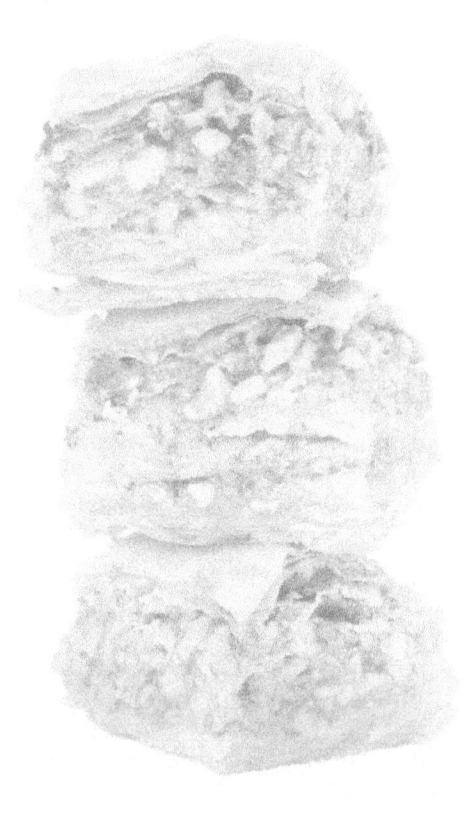

Chapter 4: The World of Turkish Snack Recipes

This chapter contains all the famous and traditional snack recipes that you have been wanting to make on your own.

4.1 Turkish Pogaça: Dumplings

Preparation Time: 25 minutes
Cooking Time: 30 minutes
Serving: 4

Ingredients:

- Yeast, two tbsp.
- Sugar, two tbsp.
- Spinach, one cup
- All-purpose flour, two cups
- Olive oil, two tbsp.
- Vegetable oil, two tbsp.
- Salt to taste
- Black pepper to taste
- Milk, two cups
- Mix cheese, two cups
- Water, as required

Instructions:

1. In a bowl mix in the yeast, sugar and two tablespoon water.
2. In a separate bowl add flour, salt, the prepared yeast mixture, and milk.
3. Knead the dough, add olive oil and then let it rise.
4. Make small round balls out of the dough.
5. Mix the feta cheese and spinach.
6. Fill these balls with the cheese and spinach mixture above.
7. Cover it with olive oil and bake for twenty to twenty-five minutes.
8. Your dish is ready to be served.

4.2 Turkish Tulimba: Fried Dough

Preparation Time: 25 minutes
Cooking Time: 20 minutes
Serving: 4

Ingredients:

- Yeast, two tbsp.
- Sugar, two tsp.
- All-purpose flour, two cups
- Olive oil, two tbsp.
- Vegetable oil, one cup

- Milk, two cups
- Eggs, two
- Water, as required
- Icing sugar, half cup

Instructions:
1. In a bowl, mix in the yeast, sugar and two tablespoon water.
2. In a separate bowl, add flour, salt, the prepared yeast mixture, and milk.
3. Knead the dough, add olive oil and then let it rise.
4. Once risen, shape it in the form of small balls leaving a hole in between.
5. Take a deep dish and add the oil in it.
6. When the oil is hot, add the prepared dough in it.
7. When the dough is golden brown dish it out.
8. Add it in icing sugar.
9. Remove the excess icing sugar.
10. Your dish is ready to be served.

4.3 Turkish Sesame Bread

Preparation Time: 25 minutes
Cooking Time: 15 minutes
Serving: 4

Ingredients:

- Yeast, two tbsp.
- Sugar, two tbsp.
- Molasses, half cup
- All-purpose flour, two cups
- Olive oil, two tbsp.
- Sesame seeds, two tbsp.
- Egg, one
- Warm water, two cups

Instructions:

1. In a bowl mix in the yeast, sugar and two tablespoon water.
2. In a separate bowl add flour, salt, the prepared yeast mixture, and milk.
3. Knead the dough, add olive oil and then let it rise.
4. Make small flat breads out of the dough.
5. Mix the molasses and sesame seeds.
6. Dip the breads in the sesame seeds mixture and place it on a baking dish.
7. Cover it with egg wash and bake for twenty to twenty-five minutes.
8. You can serve it with any side dish you prefer.
9. Your dish is ready to be served.

4.4 Turkish Kabak Tatlisi: Pumpkin Dessert

Preparation Time: 25 minutes

Cooking Time: 15 minutes

Serving: 4

Ingredients:

- Pumpkin slices, two pounds
- Sugar, two tbsp.
- Molasses, half cup

Instructions:

1. Add the pumpkin slices on the baking dish.
2. Add the molasses and sugar on top.
3. Bake for fifteen minutes.
4. When the pumpkin slices are soft enough dish out.
5. Your dish is ready to be served.

Turkish Cookbook

4.5 Turkish Sigara Borek

Preparation Time: 25 minutes

Cooking Time: 15 minutes

Serving: 4

Ingredients:
- Honey, two tbsp.
- Puff pastry dough, a pack
- Egg, one
- Yoghurt, half cup
- Sugar, two tbsp.
- Unsalted butter, two tbsp.

Instructions:
1. Mix the sugar, butter together.
2. Add two pastry sheets on top of another on a dry surface.
3. Spread little amount of the mixture all around the pastry sheet.
4. Add the leftover sheets on top.
5. Cut them into little squares.
6. Round them in the form of cigar.
7. Brush the edges of the top pastry with softened spread.
8. Take a pan and heat it well.

9. Add the pastry into the oven and cook for forty minutes.
10. Serve the borek warm.
11. Your dish is ready to be served.

4.6 Turkish Delight

Preparation Time: 25 minutes

Cooking Time: 60 minutes

Serving: 4

Ingredients:
- Cream of tartar, two tsp.
- Corn flour, three tbsp.
- Icing sugar, half cup
- Granulated sugar, half cup
- Pink food color, a pinch
- Oil, two tbsp.

Instructions:
1. In a deep pan, add the granulated sugar.
2. Let the sugar melt and then add the cream of tartar.
3. Add the corn flour and mix it for five minutes.
4. Add in the pink food color.
5. Add the mixture in a tray.

Turkish Cookbook

6. Once the mixture solidifies, cut it into small pieces.
7. Add the icing sugar on top.
8. Remove the excess sugar.
9. Your dish is ready to be served.

4.7 Turkish Śutlac

Preparation Time: 25 minutes
Cooking Time: 15 minutes
Serving: 4

Ingredients:

- Sugar, four tbsp.
- Cardamom essence, two drops
- Rice, half cup
- Milk, two cups
- Water, one cup

Instructions:

1. Add the milk in a pan.
2. Boil the milk and add the rice.
3. Add the water into the mixture.
4. Add sugar and cardamom essence.
5. Cook it for fifteen minutes.

6. When the dish thickens out.
7. Add sugar syrup on top and let it cool.
8. Your dish is ready to be served.

4.8 Turkish Churros

Preparation Time: 25 minutes
Cooking Time: 20 minutes
Serving: 4

Ingredients:
- Yeast, two tbsp.
- Sugar, two tsp.
- All-purpose flour, two cups
- Olive oil, two tbsp.
- Vegetable oil, one cup
- Milk, two cups
- Eggs, two
- Water, as required

Instructions:
1. In a bowl, mix in the yeast, sugar and two tablespoon water.
2. In a separate bowl, add flour, salt, the prepared yeast mixture, and milk.

3. Knead the dough, add olive oil and then let it rise.
4. Once risen, shape it in the form of long fingers.
5. Take a deep dish and add the oil in it.
6. When the oil is hot, add the prepared dough in it.
7. When the dough is golden brown dish it out.
8. You can serve it with any dip you desire.
9. Your dish is ready to be served.

4.9 Turkish Baklava

Preparation Time: 25 minutes

Cooking Time: 15 minutes

Serving: 4

Ingredients:

- Sugar syrup, one cup
- Puff pastry dough, a pack
- Pistachio, three tbsp.
- Clotted cream, half cup
- Sugar, two tbsp.
- Unsalted butter, two tbsp.

Instructions:
1. Add two pastry sheets on top of another on a dry surface.
2. Spread little amount of the cream all around the pastry sheet.
3. Sprinkle the finely squashed pistachios and sugar uniformly over the cream.
4. Add the leftover sheets on top.
5. Cut them into little squares.
6. Brush the edges of the top pastry with softened spread.
7. Bake the pastry until they turn golden brown.
8. Add the sugar syrup on top once the pastry is cooked.
9. Your dish is ready to be served.

4.10 Turkish Coffee

Preparation Time: 5 minutes
Cooking Time: 15 minutes
Serving: 2

Ingredients:
- Sugar, one tsp.
- Ground coffee, one tbsp.
- Water, one cup
- Ground cardamom, one tsp.

Instructions:

1. Add water, sugar, and ground cardamom in a small saucepan.
2. When the water is boiled remove the saucepan from heat.
3. Add the ground coffee and mix it.
4. Again, place the saucepan on heat.
5. When the coffee bubbles out remove from heat.
6. Pour the coffee into two cups.
7. Your dish is ready to be served.

4.11 Turkish Helva

Preparation Time: 5 minutes
Cooking Time: 15 minutes
Serving: 4

Ingredients:

- Walnuts, half cup
- Flour, two cups
- Water, two cups
- Sugar, one cup
- Butter, two tbsp.
- Pistachios, half cup

Instructions:
1. Add the butter and flour in a pan.
2. Cook it for five minutes and then when the color changes add the sugar.
3. Add the water and mix it effectively.
4. Add the walnuts and pistachios in the helva.
5. Your dish is ready to be served.

4.12 Kabak mücveri: Turkish Fritters

Preparation Time: 25 minutes
Cooking Time: 15 minutes
Serving: 4

Ingredients:
- Chopped garlic, two tsp.
- Green onions, three tbsp.
- Zucchini, two cups
- Chopped fresh dill, two tbsp.
- Vegetable oil, as required
- Cumin spice, two tbsp.
- Salt to taste
- Gram flour, two cups

- Chopped onions, two tbsp.
- Water, as required

Instructions:
1. Mix all the ingredients together.
2. Heat the oil in a large pan.
3. Make small fritters and fry them.
4. When the fritters are golden brown dish them out.
5. Serve them with your preferred dip.
6. Your dish is ready to be served.

4.13 Turkish Haydari

Preparation Time: 10 minutes

Cooking Time: 5 minutes

Serving: 4

Ingredients:
- Chopped garlic, two tsp.
- Green onions, three tbsp.
- Yoghurt, two cups
- Chopped fresh dill, two tbsp.
- Olive oil, two tbsp.
- Salt to taste

- Black pepper to taste
- Chopped tomatoes, one cup
- Chopped onions, two tbsp.

Instructions:
1. Mix all the ingredients together to form a smooth paste.
2. Serve it with bread slices or any other side dish you prefer.
3. Your dish is ready to be served.

4.14 Hummus

Preparation Time: 25 minutes
Cooking Time: 15 minutes
Serving: 4

Ingredients:
- Olive oil, two tbsp.
- Chopped garlic, two tsp.
- Cooked chickpeas, two cups
- Parsley, as required

Instructions:
1. Blend the olive oil, garlic, and chickpeas.
2. When the blend is smooth enough add it in a bowl.

3. Add the olive oil on top.
4. Add parsley on top.
5. Your dish is ready to be served.

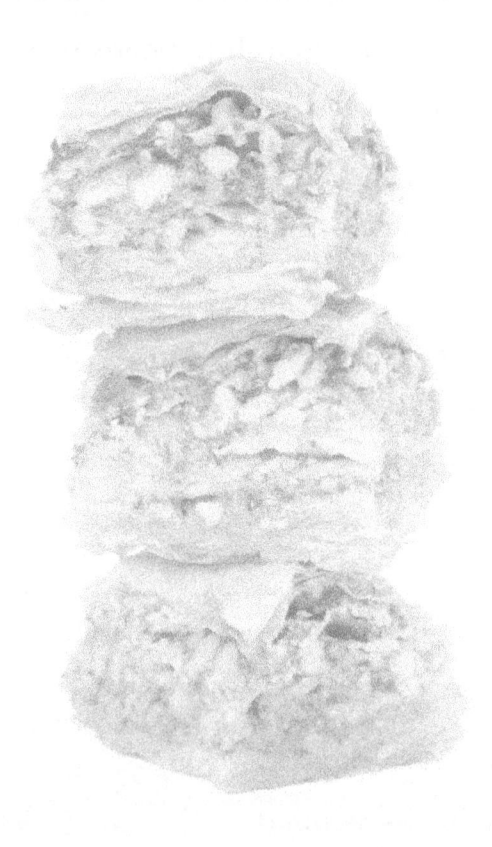

Chapter 5: The World of Turkish Vegetarian Recipes

This chapter contains all the famous and traditional vegetarian recipes that you have been wanting to make on your own.

5.1 Yaprak Sarma

Preparation Time: 25 minutes
Cooking Time: 5 minutes
Serving Size: 4-6

Ingredients:

- Shredded green cabbage, two cups
- Cooked bulgar, two cups
- Sliced red bell pepper, one cup
- Shredded carrots, one cup
- Sliced yellow bell pepper, one cup
- Green onions, a quarter cup
- Parsley, a quarter cup
- Salt and pepper to taste
- Sesame seeds, half cup
- Vine leaves, as required

- Thread, as required

Instructions:
1. Add all of the ingredients to a large bowl.
2. Drizzle your desired amount of the sesame seeds over the mixture.
3. Toss the mixture until well combined.
4. Add the mixture on the vine leaves and roll it in the form of kebabs.
5. Tie it with thread so it does not fall out.
6. Let the sarma cook with the help of steam.
7. Place them on a pan full of boiling water for fifteen minutes.
8. Remove the thread from each sarma before serving.
9. Your dish is ready to be served.

5.2 Enginar Kalbi

Preparation Time: 25 minutes
Cooking Time: 30 minutes
Serving: 4

Ingredients:
- Mix Turkish spice, two tbsp.
- Chopped garlic, two tsp.

- Green onions, three tbsp.
- Chopped artichokes, two cups
- Chopped fresh dill, two tbsp.
- Vegetable oil, half cup
- Salt to taste
- Black pepper to taste
- Bread crumbs, two tbsp.
- Chopped onions, two tbsp.
- Tomato puree, two cups

Instructions:
1. In a bowl, add the minced artichokes, chopped garlic, onions, fresh dill, spices, and bread crumbs together.
2. Mix the above ingredients to form a fine and smooth structure.
3. Make small round ball like structures.
4. In a pan, add the oil and heat it.
5. When the oil is heated enough add the balls and fry them all over.
6. When the balls are golden brown in color dish them out.
7. In a pan add the tomato puree and place the balls in it.
8. Once the gravy is cooked switch off the stove.
9. Your dish is ready to be served.

5.3 Barbunya: Turkish Beans

Preparation Time: 25 minutes

Cooking Time: 40 minutes

Serving: 4

Ingredients:
- Mix Turkish spice, two tbsp.
- Chopped garlic, two tsp.
- Green onions, three tbsp.
- Beans, two cups
- Vegetable stock, half cup
- Chopped fresh dill, two tbsp.
- Vegetable oil, half cup
- Salt to taste
- Black pepper to taste
- Parsley, two tbsp.
- Tomatoes, one cup
- Chopped onions, two tbsp.

Instructions:
10. Add the oil in a deep pan.
11. Add the chopped onions when the oil is hot.
12. When the onions are soft enough add the garlic into it.

13. Add in the tomatoes and all the spices.
14. Add in the beans and mix it for ten minutes.
15. Add in the vegetable stock.
16. Let the beans simmer for thirty minutes.
17. In the end add the green onions and parsley and dish out.
18. Your dish is ready to be served.

5.4 Carrot Balls and Yoghurt

Preparation Time: 25 minutes
Cooking Time: 15 minutes
Serving: 4

Ingredients:
- Chopped garlic, two tsp.
- Green onions, three tbsp.
- Carrots, two cups
- Chopped fresh dill, two tbsp.
- Vegetable oil, as required
- Cumin spice, two tbsp.
- Salt to taste
- Gram flour, two cups
- Chopped onions, two tbsp.
- Water, as required

- Yoghurt, one cup
- Bread slices, as required

Instructions:
1. Mix all the ingredients together.
2. Heat the oil in a large pan.
3. Make small balls and fry them.
4. When the balls are golden brown dish them out.
5. Serve them with yoghurt and bread.
6. Your dish is ready to be served.

5.5 Firin Sebze

Preparation Time: 25 minutes

Cooking Time: 40 minutes

Serving: 4

Ingredients:
- Mix Turkish spice, two tbsp.
- Chopped garlic, two tsp.
- Green onions, three tbsp.
- Mix vegetables, two cups
- Chopped fresh dill, two tbsp.
- Vegetable oil, half cup

- Salt to taste
- Black pepper to taste
- Parsley, two tbsp.
- Tomatoes, one cup
- Chopped onions, two tbsp.

Instructions:
1. Add the oil in a deep pan.
2. Add the chopped onions when the oil is hot.
3. When the onions are soft enough, add the garlic into it.
4. Add in the tomatoes and all the spices.
5. Add in the vegetables and mix it for ten minutes.
6. Let the vegetables simmer for thirty minutes.
7. In the end add the green onions and parsley and dish out.
8. Your dish is ready to be served.

5.6 Kuru Fasulye: Turkish Bean Stew

Preparation Time: 25 minutes

Cooking Time: 40 minutes

Serving: 4

Ingredients:
- Mix Turkish spice, two tbsp.
- Chopped garlic, two tsp.
- Green onions, three tbsp.
- Beans, two cups
- Bean stock, three cups
- Chopped fresh dill, two tbsp.
- Vegetable oil, half cup
- Salt to taste
- Black pepper to taste
- Parsley, two tbsp.
- Tomatoes, one cup
- Chopped onions, two tbsp.

Instructions:
1. Add the oil in a deep pan.
2. Add the chopped onions when the oil is hot.
3. When the onions are soft enough, add the garlic into it.

4. Add in the tomatoes and all the spices.
5. Add in the beans and mix it for ten minutes.
6. Add in the bean stock.
7. Let the beans simmer for thirty minutes.
8. In the end, add the green onions and parsley and dish out.
9. Your dish is ready to be served.

5.7 Corba: Turkish Soup

Preparation Time: 25 minutes

Cooking Time: 40 minutes

Serving: 4

Ingredients:
- Mix Turkish spice, two tbsp.
- Chopped garlic, two tsp.
- Green onions, three tbsp.
- Mix vegetables, two cups
- Water, two cups
- Corn flour, two tbsp.
- Cooked bulgar, one cup
- Chopped fresh dill, two tbsp.
- Vegetable oil, half cup
- Salt to taste

- Black pepper to taste
- Parsley, two tbsp.
- Tomatoes, one cup
- Chopped onions, two tbsp.

Instructions:

11. Add the oil in a deep pan.
12. Add the chopped onions when the oil is hot.
13. When the onions are soft enough, add the garlic into it.
14. Add in the tomatoes and all the spices.
15. Add in the vegetables and mix it for ten minutes.
16. Let the vegetables simmer for thirty minutes.
17. Add in the water and cook for five minutes.
18. Add in the corn flour and cooked bulgar.
19. In the end add the green onions and parsley and dish out.
20. Your dish is ready to be served.

5.8 Zeytinyagli Taze Fasulye

Preparation Time: 25 minutes

Cooking Time: 40 minutes

Serving: 4

Ingredients:

- Mix Turkish spice, two tbsp.
- Chopped garlic, two tsp.
- Green onions, three tbsp.
- Green beans, two cups
- Chopped fresh dill, two tbsp.
- Vegetable oil, half cup
- Salt to taste
- Black pepper to taste
- Parsley, two tbsp.
- Tomatoes, one cup
- Chopped onions, two tbsp.

Instructions:
1. Add the oil in a deep pan.
2. Add the chopped onions when the oil is hot.
3. When the onions are soft enough, add the garlic into it.
4. Add in the tomatoes and all the spices.
5. Add in the green beans and mix it for ten minutes.
6. Let the green beans simmer for thirty minutes.
7. In the end add the green onions and parsley and dish out.
8. Your dish is ready to be served.

5.9 Dolma

Preparation Time: 25 minutes

Cooking Time: 5 minutes

Serving Size: 4-6

Ingredients:
- Cooked bulgar, two cups
- Sliced red bell pepper, one cup
- Shredded carrots, one cup
- Green onions, a quarter cup
- Parsley, a quarter cup
- Salt and pepper to taste
- Sesame seeds, half cup
- Vine leaves, as required
- Thread, as required

Instructions:
1. Add all of the ingredients to a large bowl.
2. Drizzle your desired amount of the sesame seeds over the mixture.
3. Toss the mixture until well combined.
4. Add the mixture on the vine leaves and roll it in the form of kebabs.
5. Tie it with thread so it does not fall out.
6. Let the dolma cook with the help of steam.

Turkish Cookbook

7. Place them on a pan full of boiling water for fifteen minutes.
8. Remove the thread from each dolma before serving.
9. Your dish is ready to be served.

5.10 Nohutlu Pilav: Turkish Rice with Chickpeas

Preparation Time: 25 minutes
Cooking Time: 40 minutes
Serving: 4

Ingredients:
- Mix Turkish spice, two tbsp.
- Chopped garlic, two tsp.
- Green onions, three tbsp.
- Chickpeas, two cups
- Rice, three cups
- Chopped fresh dill, two tbsp.
- Vegetable oil, half cup
- Salt to taste
- Black pepper to taste
- Parsley, two tbsp.
- Tomatoes, one cup
- Chopped onions, two tbsp.

Instructions:

1. Add the oil in a deep pan.
2. Add the chopped onions when the oil is hot.
3. When the onions are soft enough, add the garlic into it.
4. Add in the tomatoes and all the spices.
5. Add in the chickpeas and mix it for ten minutes.
6. Add in the rice and let the stew simmer for thirty minutes.
7. In the end add the green onions and parsley and dish out.
8. Your dish is ready to be served.

5.11 Turkish Stuffed Peppers

Preparation Time: 25 minutes
Cooking Time: 15 minutes
Serving: 4

Ingredients:

- Olive oil, two tbsp.
- Chopped garlic, two tsp.
- Green onions, three tbsp.
- Bell peppers, four
- Zucchini, two cups
- Chopped fresh dill, two tbsp.
- Vegetable oil, two tbsp.

- Salt to taste
- Black pepper to taste
- Bulgar, one cup
- Mixed cheese, one cup
- Chopped onions, two tbsp.

Instructions:

10. Mix all the ingredients together in a bowl.
11. Cut the bell peppers in half.
12. Remove the seeds from inside.
13. Stuff the formed mixture into the bell peppers.
14. Place the bell peppers on a baking dish.
15. Add the cheese on top.
16. Drizzle oil on top.
17. Bake for fifteen minutes.
18. Your dish is ready to be served.

5.12 Turkish Batrik

Preparation Time: 25 minutes

Cooking Time: 5 minutes

Serving Size: 4-6

Ingredients:

- Shredded green cabbage, two cups
- Cooked bulgar, two cups
- Sliced red bell pepper, one cup
- Shredded carrots, one cup
- Sliced yellow bell pepper, one cup
- Green onions, a quarter cup
- Honey, two tbsp.
- Parsley, a quarter cup
- Salt and pepper to taste
- Sesame seeds, half cup
- Tomato dressing, one cup

Instructions:
1. Add all of the salad ingredients to a large bowl.
2. Drizzle your desired amount of the sesame seeds over the salad.
3. Add the tomato dressing on top.
4. Toss the salad until well combined.
5. Your dish is ready to be served.

5.13 Cig Kofte

Preparation Time: 25 minutes
Cooking Time: 30 minutes

Serving: 4

Ingredients:

- Mix Turkish spice, two tbsp.
- Chopped garlic, two tsp.
- Green onions, three tbsp.
- Mixed vegetables, two cups
- Chopped fresh dill, two tbsp.
- Vegetable oil, half cup
- Salt to taste
- Black pepper to taste
- Chopped onions, two tbsp.

Instructions:

1. In a bowl, add the mixed vegetables, chopped garlic, onions, fresh dill, and spices together.
2. Mix the above ingredients to form a fine and smooth structure in a blender.
3. Freeze the mixture above in a tight container.
4. Cut out bite sizes when the mixture freezes completely.
5. Your dish is ready to be served.

Conclusion

The Turkish cooking is a blend; it took the best nourishments anyone in the Empire could make. It likewise offered back a portion of these food sources. Great Turkish food is restricted, it comes from a particular spot and duplicating it in different locales is not acceptable. Some of the recipes with time have changed and have become something different. The cooking cycle develops and adjusts to various districts.

Balkans was a basic and significant piece of Ottoman Empire for a couple of a good centuries. It is entirely sensible to see its culinary effects on the area. Moreover, it is likewise basic to comprehend the qualities of strict networks which described what Balkans eat, for example Muslims and Christians.

We have discussed 77 different recipes comprising of breakfast, lunch, dinner, snack, and vegetarian recipes. You can easily make all these recipes at home without any problem with the detailed ingredient list and easy to follow instructions. So, now you can cook easily like a professional Turkish chef on your own.

Turkish Cookbook

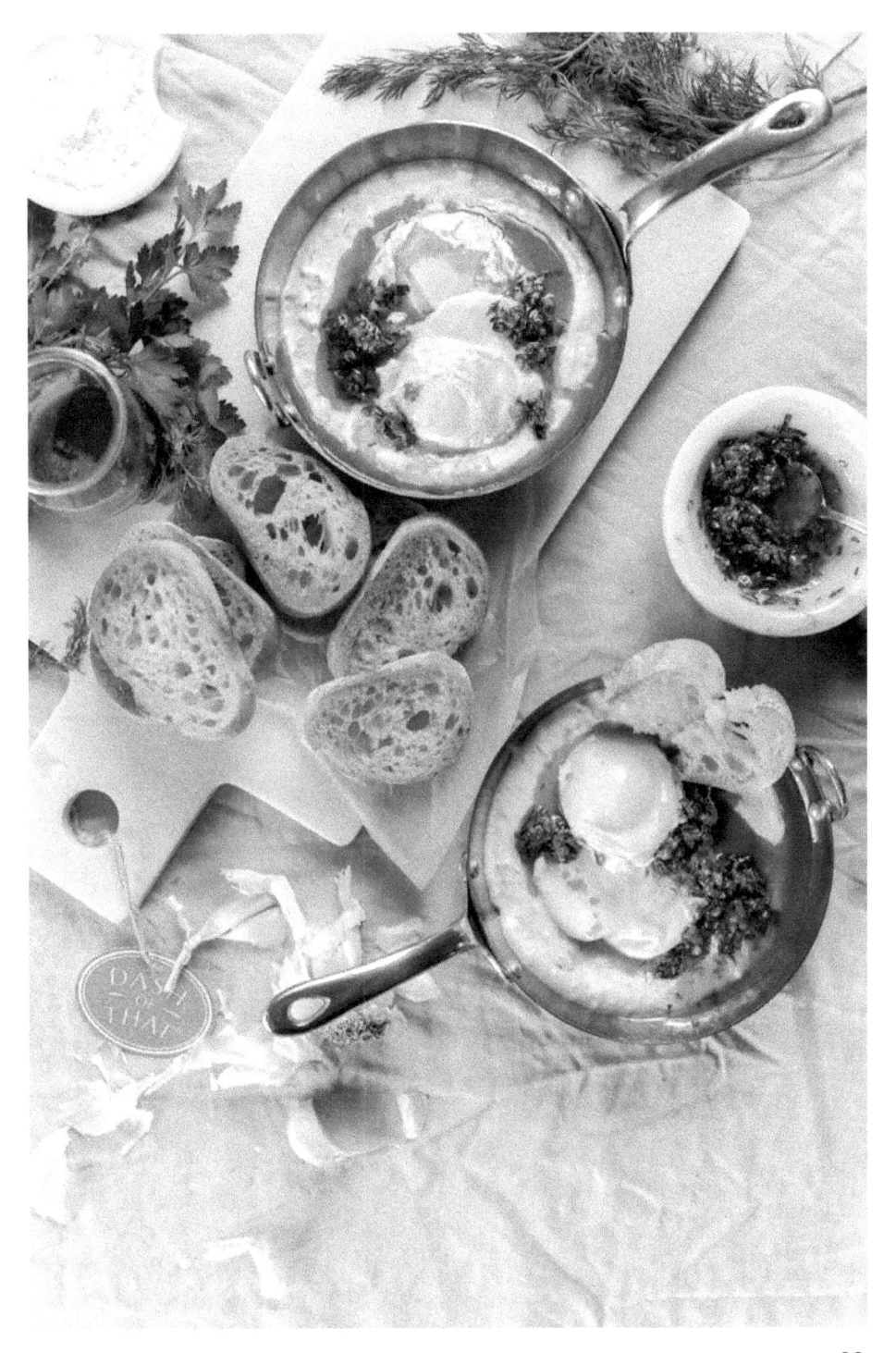

Turkish Cookbook

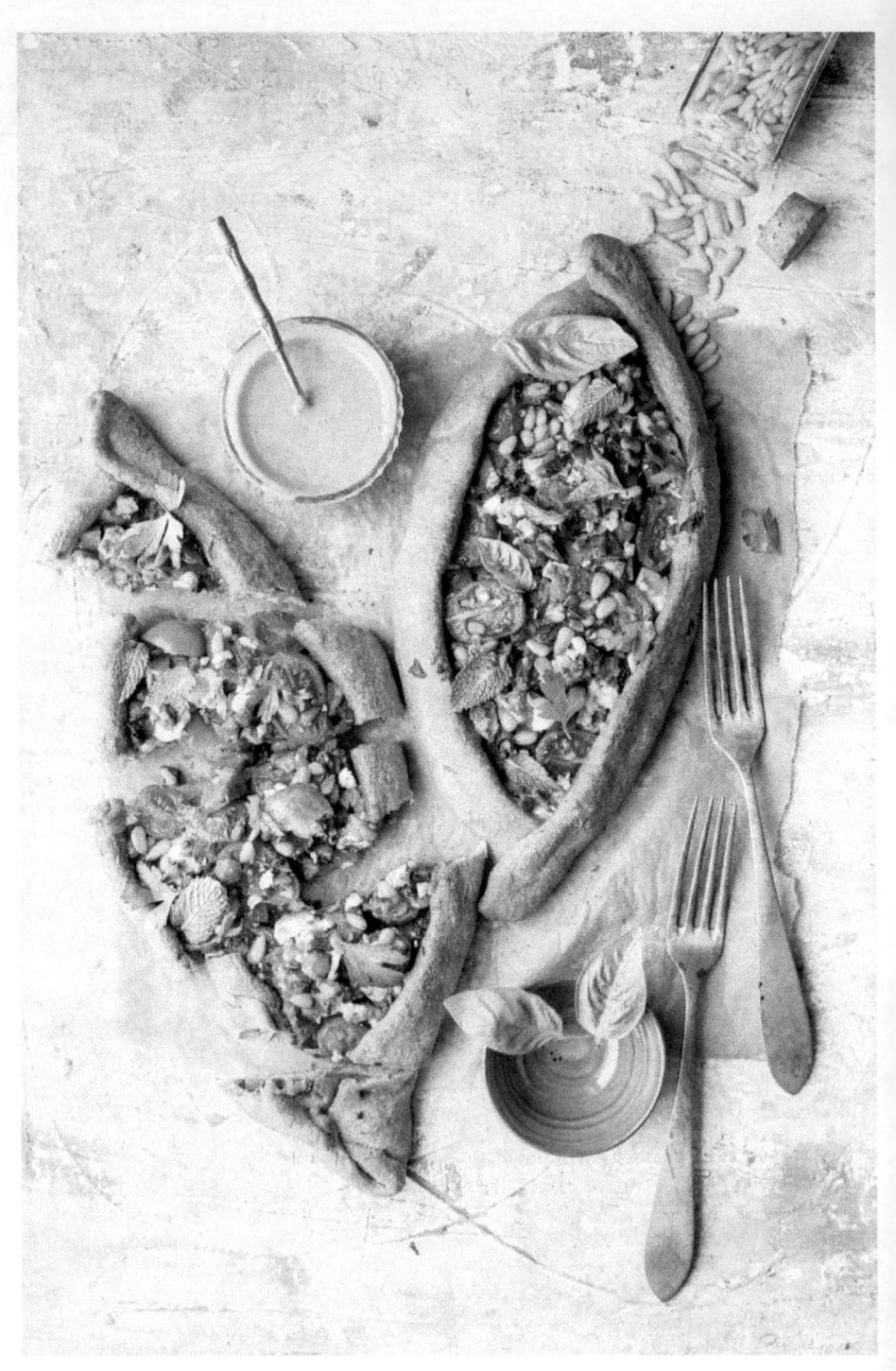

Lightning Source UK Ltd.
Milton Keynes UK
UKHW021836220621
385995UK00002B/218

9 781802 764185